WHAT YOU

BLOOD

TELLS YOU…..

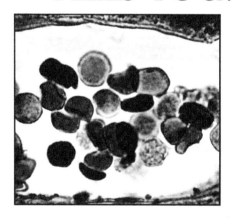

ENERGETIC,
NUTRITIONAL
ANSWERS FOR CHANGE

JOSEPH R. SCOGNA, JR.
& KATHY M. SCOGNA

Special thanks to Kalli M. Scogna for typing and keeping this on track, and Rachel Lickter for proof reading and many helpful suggestions.

What Your Blood Tells You –Energetic, Nutritional Answers for Change

Originally published in the USA as *The Blood Works* by Joseph R. Scogna, Jr., 1980. Revised, edited and compiled by Kathy M. Scogna as What Your Blood Tells You....2005. Life Energy Publications * www.LifeEnergyResearch.com

Available as a Kindle e-Book

Notice: This work reflects the research of Joseph R. Scogna, Jr., nutritionists and homeopathic physicians worldwide. It is not a medical manual nor should it be used to diagnose diseases or prescribe medicine or drugs. Based on nutritional research, the nutrients and herbs are provided for reference and educational purposes so that adults can make informed decisions about their health. The reader should be aware that any substance (food or medicine) may cause allergic reactions in some people. The reader is urged to evaluate his or her health status and if disease, poor health, illness or continuing symptoms, however minor, are present, he or she should seek the proper health practitioner.

What Your Blood Tells You: Energetic, Nutritional Answers for Change
Includes index
1.   Blood Chemistry Tests 2. Nutrition 3. Self help
I. Joseph R. Scogna, Jr. author II. Kathy M. Scogna author, editor III. Title

ISBN- 13: 978-1497465442
ISBN-10: 1497465443

Contents

Introduction   5

Major Organs and Glands   6

Blood Chemistry Tests   7

How to Use this Book   8

1. Calcium (Ca), serum   9
2. Phosphorus (P)   11
3. Blood Urea Nitrogen (BUN)   13
4. Glucose   15
5. Uric Acid, serum   18
6. Total Cholesterol, serum   20
7. Total Protein   22
8. Albumin, serum   24
9. Bilirubin, total   26
10. Alkaline Phosphatase (ALP), serum   28
11. Lactate Dehydrogenase (LDH), serum   30
12. Asparte Aminotransferase AST
    (formerly SGOT)   32
13. Total Globulins   34
14. Albumin/Globulin (A/G) ratio   36
15. Sodium (Na), serum   38
16. Potassium (K) serum   40
17. Chloride (Cl). Serum   42
18. Carbon Dioxide (CO_2), serum   44
19. Creatinine ($C_4H_7ON_3$), serum   46
20. Iron (Fe), serum   48
21. BUN/Creatinine Ratio   50
22. Triglycerides, serum   52
23. Alanine Aminotransferase (ALT)
    (formerly SGPT)   55
24. Thyroxine (T_4)   57
25. Complete Blood Count (CBC)   59

References   64

Index   65

(For alphabetical listing, see page 4)

Alphabetical Listing of Tests

Alanine Aminotransferase (ALT) (Formerly SGPT)	55
Albumin, serum	24
Albumin/Globulin (A/G) ratio	36
Alkaline Phosphatase (ALP), serum	28
Asparte Aminotransferase AST (formerly SGOT)	32
Bilirubin, total	26
Blood Urea Nitrogen (BUN)	13
BUN/Creatinine Ratio	50
Calcium (Ca), serum	9
Carbon Dioxide (CO_2), serum	44
Chloride (Cl). Serum	42
Cholesterol, serum, Total	20
Complete Blood Count (CBC)	59
Creatinine ($C_4H_7ON_3$), serum	46
Globulins, Total	34
Glucose	15
Iron (Fe), serum	48
Lactate Dehydrogenase (LDH), serum	30
Phosphorus (P)	11
Potassium (K) serum	40
Protein, Total	22
Sodium (Na), serum	38
Thyroxine (T_4)	57
Triglycerides, serum	52
Uric Acid, serum	18

Introduction

What is your blood cholesterol number? How are your triglycerides? If you are a weight lifter, your creatinine number will have special significance.

Have you ever wondered what vitamins, minerals, juices, essential oils, herbs or other nutrients and foods might adjust these numbers?

To anyone interested in their own nutritional health and symptoms, these are common questions. It seems we all have an innate desire to know what makes our body perform the miracle it does. This has led many searchers to delve into various realms of science seeking the answers.

The simple fact is that <u>the body is a machine</u>, and in its smallest sense, the blood <u>is</u> the body. The blood is a micro-universe. As the blood circulates through our veins and arteries, it carries oxygen and nutrients to our cells and tissues. When the metabolic processes are completed, it miraculously removes the waste products and carbon dioxide from the cells for transport and disposal. The blood is replete with all the materials and ingredients necessary to build and sustain us. Everything is in our blood to make us what we are today and to shape us into what we will be tomorrow.

Of course, a lack of vital nutrients or an excess of poisons affects the role our blood plays. If we aren't eating wholesome and nutritious foods, or if we are under too much stress at work or at home, or if we live in close proximity to industrial sites, nuclear power plants, or electronic pollution such as computers and cell phones, our body and its small but most vital part, the blood, will be affected.

While no two individuals are alike, we do indeed share the same humanoid blueprint – all of us under the sun depend on blood.

Perhaps in the future, men and women will possess bionically constructed android bodies with few moving parts that can exist on alternating current and occasional lube jobs. But here, in the present, we must pay tribute to that marvelous, rich liquid which courses through the body by the microsecond to keep us alive – we must learn all we can about how *the blood works*.

—JRS, JR.

The Major Organs and Glands

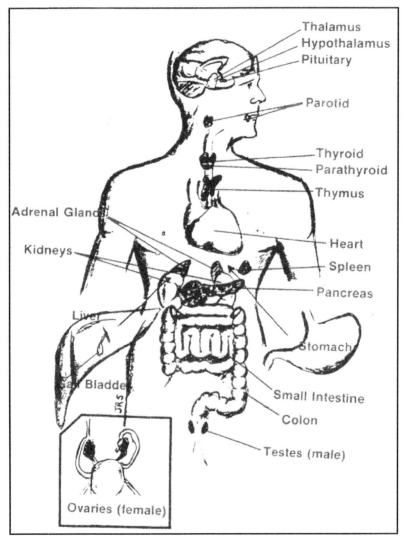

Blood Chemistry Tests

The laboratory scientist uses blood evaluations that relate to time, presence, and color. In other words, chemical reagents are employed to detect the <u>presence</u> of certain properties of the blood by the amount of <u>time</u> it takes to turn a certain <u>color</u>. This is an oversimplification but, along with microscopic screening, is the basic logic used to determine blood values.

Blood values vary from lab to lab and it is the writer's viewpoint and the belief of many other researchers that the values vary from person to person – perhaps far more so than is now realized. The efficacy of the blood test does not, as such, rely on the <u>standard</u> values but the <u>change</u> of reading. If the rate of change exceeds the accepted standards there is usually an obvious problem, but we can use the blood test to observe electrolytes, glucose and increases and decreases in enzymatic activity. This action will reveal trends that can be observed and used as a guideline to further research.

Among nutritional researchers, it is a major point of controversy as to how much significance should be placed on the readings we get from a standard blood chemistry test. While blood laboratories publish their normal ranges in wide variances, pioneers in the field of nutrition tend to narrow the margin considerably. Any given lab may consider the cholesterol reading of a patient in the "normal range" while two separate research scientists will differ as to whether the reading is <u>too</u> <u>high</u> or <u>too</u> <u>low</u>! Thus, the lack of a true standard makes a single blood test subject to broad interpretation unless it is grossly off the mark and, even then, the sometimes-fickle body processes frustrate the researcher.

There are many other factors, including personal health profile and family genetic predisposition that should be taken into account. Perhaps more significant is the type of food eaten for several days previous to blood being drawn—was it sugary doughnuts, daily prime ribs of beef, or salads and vegetables?

Blood test results are produced by machine. The SMA, developed in 1967, and the SMAC, released in 1973, are the main instruments (SMAC = Sequential Multiple Analyzer + Computer), which run colorimetric studies on the electric potential and enzymatic activities of the various properties of the blood. A good reason why two or more tests should be run – man and his machines are not flawless! Needless upset and mistaken "health hazard" or even faulty "clean bill of health" reports have resulted from the mishandling of specimens, machine failure, and just plain human error. The person being tested should always get a second opinion before embarking on a suggested program, either by corroboration of evidence by other testing methods, such as hair mineral analysis or urine tests, or a follow up blood chemistry evaluation.

How to Use this Book

Depending upon the state in which you live, many outpatient labs offer blood screenings without requiring a prescription and this book can be used for your own evaluation. Or, if you are a patient of a practitioner and are interested in your body, and would like to take responsibility for your own health and symptoms, make a note of your blood chemistry numbers the next time your practitioner orders one.

Each chapter lists:

- The laboratory norms and nutritional research norms (these lab norms may vary by location).
- Technical explanation of the item.
- Remedies for the highs and lows. Remedies can be taken as tea, tincture, flower essence, essential oil, pill form or homeopathic. (The homeopathic or the electromagnetic frequency of the remedy is preferred. See *Homeopathy Revisited*.)
- Visit www.LifeEnergyResearch.com, complete a holistic questionnaire, then access SAFonline for energetic, nutritional suggestions for YOU, based on your answers and the sequence of numbers.
- Find an SAF practitioner; read about your sequence of numbers in SAF Simplified.

The nutritional information provided here, while not intended for diagnosis or prescription, can be an extremely helpful guide for practitioners and the nutritional enthusiast.

1. Calcium (Ca), serum

Norms:

Laboratory	9 – 11.0 mg/100 ml
Nutritional Research	9.7 – 10.7 mg/100 ml

Calcium is one of the most important elements in the body. It is a light mineral and yet it gives our body its firmness and rigidity. Calcium is essential for the formation of the bones and the teeth.

The parathyroid gland is its chief regulator and makes it possible to keep calcium ionized in the blood stream. These calcium particles revolve around the body in constant motion to stabilize the acid/alkaline balance of the body, as well as to promote lactation, activate enzymes, and to facilitate the function of the muscles, nerves, and heart. Vitamin D works with the parathyroid gland and calcium to expedite charged calcium from the bones to the tissues and cross the membrane system of the body. This action takes place to prevent acid conditions from developing in <u>any</u> area of the body. When this ability of the body wears down, the system begins to lose pliability and the stony indurations of arthritis, rheumatism, arteriosclerosis, and heart disease develop.

When the blood reading of calcium is higher than the accepted health standard, there is an imbalance in the acid-alkaline balance of the blood. The imbalance is in the calcium-magnesium ratio causing poor digestion of fats, starches, and proteins; in this case there may be a high alkaline condition in the small intestine.

The remedy for high calcium is to provide the electromagnetic frequencies or substances of: magnesium, digestive enzymes, oat straw, alfalfa, licorice, nettle, red clover, pulsatilla, and chamomile.

When the blood reading of calcium is lower that the accepted health standard, the activation of certain enzymes of fatty acids will be greatly hampered. This slows electron transmission throughout the body and affects the nervous system's ability to "keep the power on" so to speak. There may be a feeling of being out of balance. The deficiency symptoms are dental caries, rickets, tetany, hyperirritability, excessive bleeding, and heart palpitations.

The remedy for low calcium is to supply the electromagnetic frequencies or substances of: ionized calcium, vitamin D, lipase, amylase, and protease, essential fatty acids, spinach, extra complete proteins, milk, whey, carrot juice, nettle, and skullcap.

For customized Energetic, Nutritional Answers:
Go to: www.LifeEnergyResearch.com
- Click "questionnaires." Complete Stress-120 Questionnaire or SAF-120 Questionnaire and receive your chain of numbers.
- Find a Remedy. Access SAFonline and use one or several Interpretations: Juices, Herbs, Homeopathics, Glandulars, Vita Coordinator, Essential Oils, Flower Essences, Chinese Herbs and many more to find the items unique to your chain and your issues.
- Find an SAF practitioner; read about your chain in *SAF Simplified*.

2. Phosphorus (P)

Norms:

Laboratory	**2.7 – 4.5 mg/100 ml**
Nutritional Research	**3.1 – 3.5 mg/100 ml**

Like calcium, phosphorus depends heavily on vitamin D and the parathyroid gland to regulate its function. The phosphorus compound adenosine triphosphate (ATP) and phosphocreatine are the chief sources of muscle energy during muscle contractions, which includes the heart muscle. Phosphorus is essential in teeth and gum health and in the delicate operation of waste disposal by the kidney and intestine. Excess amounts may be excreted as a result of improper energy conversion as in situations of hypoglycemia and diabetes.

Phosphorus is a trivalent anion (negatively charged), which regulates the entire spectrum of elements in coordination with the acid-alkaline balance of the body. It regulates and aligns minerals, enzymes, sugars, proteins, and fats in a coordinated attempt to adjust the present body condition with the electrical blueprint of the genetic code. In other words, phosphorus is the most important watch guard of systemic equilibrium.

When the blood reading of phosphorus is higher than the accepted health standard, there may be a change in appetite, muscle contractions, or bone growth. A high blood reading of phosphorus hints at the probability of slowed chemical electrical reaction in digestion where the element may be inert or on the toxic side of the balance. This situation indicates a build up of phosphorus ions and the rapid development of phosphorus-bound compounds.

Phosphorus is stimulated by electrical devices, such as television, x-ray, microwaves and other electronic stressors.

The remedy for high phosphorus is to supply the electromagnetic frequencies or substances of: kidney, hydrochloric acid (HCI), ammonium chloride, folic acid, zinc, sulfur-bearing amino acids Methionine and lysine, and the essential nitrogen-bearing nucleic acids, ginseng, cranberry, and dandelion.

Evaluate the electronic stressors in life.

When the blood reading of phosphorus is lower than the accepted health standard, the digestion of sugars, as well as the utilization of energy for muscle strength and power, is greatly diminished. In severe cases with calcium/phosphorus deficiency, there may be weight loss, weakness, retarded growth or disturbed tooth or bone development such as rickets. There may be physical fatigue or nervous disorders. In this situation, compounds containing orthophosphoric acid may be of value. There may be an upset in the ability to convert glucose into energy due to mental stress.

The remedy for low phosphorus is to supply the electromagnetic frequencies or substances of: pancreatic enzymes, thiamin (vitamin B1), B complex vitamins, folic acid, B2, B3, and orthophosphoric acid. Homeopathy: Sulfur, Antimony, Sepia.

Organic foods rich in protein are needed: meat, fish, poultry, eggs, whole grains, seeds and nuts.

Evaluate the mental stressors with SAF Stress-120 Questionnaire and *SAF Simplified*.

3. Blood Urea Nitrogen (BUN)

Norms:

Laboratory	**7 – 20 mg/100 ml**
Nutritional Research	**13-17 mg/100 ml**

The blood urea nitrogen (BUN) is an important test. While its function is basically to monitor and search for any signs of liver or kidney disease or malnutrition, the BUN can also be called on to give some insights into whether the body had a severe shock, was dehydrated, or was undergoing some excessive protein breakdown. When the BUN is elevated, it is usually due to an increase in the backup of urea into the blood stream. There are several reasons why this may happen including the excessive use of different types of antibiotics. The BUN is a good indicator of how well the glands dispose of their nitrogenous wastes by way of the liver. In other words, the liver, being the last depot of all of the metabolic waste released by the organs after normal activity has taken place, is a gauge of waste disposal efficiency.

When the BUN is higher then the accepted health standard, it is usually a sign of an infection causing massive releases of nitrogenous protein bodies, which are too much for the kidneys to process all at once. High BUN has been found in diabetics and those suffering from dehydration.

The remedy for high BUN is to supply the electromagnetic frequencies or substances of: the kidney, pituitary, thyroid, thymus, pancreas and adrenal glands; magnesium, B6, potassium/sodium citrate, amino acids Methionine and lysine; vitamin K, cranberry, and dandelion.

Increase distilled or reverse osmosis water consumption. (Body weight ÷ 2 = # of ounces to drink)

Detoxification formula needed.

When the BUN is lower than the accepted health standard, in extreme cases it indicates the presence of severe liver disease, malnutrition, or possibly over-hydration.

Be advised that during pregnancy, BUN naturally decreases.

The remedy for low BUN is to supply the electromagnetic frequencies or substances of: the liver; potassium; vitamin E, vitamin A, and dandelion leaf.

For customized Energetic, Nutritional Answers:
Go to: www.LifeEnergyResearch.com
- Click "questionnaires." Complete Stress-120 Questionnaire or SAF-120 Questionnaire and receive your chain of numbers.
- Find a Remedy. Access SAFonline and use one or several Interpretations: Juices, Herbs, Homeopathics, Glandulars, Vita Coordinator, Essential Oils, Flower Essences, Chinese Herbs and many more to find the items unique to your chain and your issues.
- Find an SAF practitioner; read about your chain in *SAF Simplified*.

4. Glucose

Norms:

Laboratory   **70-115 mg/100 ml**
Nutritional Research   **85-100 mg/100 ml**

Glucose is the most vital substance in the body system. Every organ needs it but the most vital organs are the anterior pituitary, the adrenal cortex and medulla, the thyroid, the gonads (testes or ovaries), and most especially the <u>brain</u>. Glucose ($C_6 H_{12} O_6$) is the ultimate statement of carbohydrate breakdown. Interlocked within its formulas are the secrets of energy and youth.

The organs use this substance as a springboard for energy. Without it, the body's systems rapidly deteriorate and lose precious energy-producing capabilities. All functions are at a standstill without the presence of glucose and its enzymes. Glucose is converted from disaccharides and polysaccharides in the small intestine following digestion. It is taken directly into the portal vein of the liver, where glucose is converted into glycogen. It is stored and released as needed for energy. Glucose is found in the blood plasma.

Conditions of too high or too low blood sugar require a variety of actions, which include the monitoring of insulin by the Islets of Langerhans, exercise, and finding and working on the stress, fear, emotional upsets, and shock factors.

Life itself is the final monitor of glucose usage. The action of glucose in the tissue is an intricate interplay between carbon, hydrogen, and oxygen. The resulting explosions of glucoside force, when ignited by ATP (Adenosine triphosphate), cause the formation of the following:

1. *the solid* – **fat**
2. *the liquid* – **water (H_2O)**
3. *the gas* – **carbon dioxide (CO_2)**

When the glucose level is higher than the accepted health standard, the individual's body is becoming flooded with end product (sugar) and ignition is becoming very scarce. When glucose is beyond saturation in the blood stream, the function of the organs show a decreased usage of minerals while at the same time a more rapid oxidation of healthy tissue. This does not necessarily depict a case of diabetes, but may show hyperglycemia, which if not controlled may lead to diabetes. Note: Only a licensed practitioner should make such a diagnosis.

The remedy for high glucose is to supply the electromagnetic frequencies or substances of: hypothalamus, brain, liver, pancreas, thymus, pituitary, gonads, adrenal glands, B Complex vitamins, garlic, ginseng, licorice, apples, fenugreek, blueberry leaf tea, and ylang ylang.

Find and process the mental stressors (fear, shock, stress).

Increase protein intake, low-fat, low-carbohydrate diet with only whole grains and vegetables.

When the blood reading of glucose is lower than the accepted health standard, hypoglycemia may be suspected. All organs use glucose more rapidly when there is a scarcity of the product. The shortage may be due to high protein and low carbohydrate foods leading to impaired digestion and very little raw material for glucose production.

If the blood glucose fluctuates (up one hour, down the next) perhaps too many simple carbohydrates are being eaten, such as white sugar, white flour, cakes and cookies. The fact that most daily diets consist of almost 40% fat attributes to the increase in cases of hypoglycemia. Fat blocks, stalls, and delays electron transfer. Fat is a favorite food for our high-strung society because it temporarily delays the high voltage stress we are experiencing today. But, the fatty insulation clogs vital electric channels and inhibits essential body processes. If the present rate of electronic pollution and stress continue their upward spiral and the American diet of fat and protein does not alter, be assured that the rate of diabetes and hypoglycemia in this country will rise even faster in the future than it has in the past!

In the case of hypoglycemia, the idea is to restore energy to its proper direction, toward the individual instead of away. This is accomplished by consuming high-powered nutrition while removing the fat barriers.

The remedy for low glucose is to supply the electromagnetic frequencies or substances of: hypothalamus, brain, pancreas, thymus, anterior and posterior pituitary, testes or ovaries, adrenal glands; calcium, magnesium, B3 (niacin), B complex vitamins to include B1, B2, B6, B12, vitamin C, tryptophan (or 5-HTP), lipase, protease, valerian, passiflora, yellow dock, ginseng, red clover, rose essential oil.

Dietary changes to contain only complex carbohydrate foods and complete proteins. No white sugar, white flour, artificial sweeteners or ingredients.

Frequent saunas are suggested to aid detoxification, but only if heat does not aggravate the drop in blood sugar.

For customized Energetic, Nutritional Answers:
Go to: www.LifeEnergyResearch.com

- Click "questionnaires." Complete Stress-120 Questionnaire or SAF-120 Questionnaire and receive your chain of numbers.
- Find a Remedy. Access SAFonline and use one or several Interpretations: Juices, Herbs, Homeopathics, Glandulars, Vita Coordinator, Essential Oils, Flower Essences, Chinese Herbs and many more to find the items unique to your chain and your issues.
- Find an SAF practitioner; read about your chain in *SAF Simplified.*

5. Uric Acid, serum

Norms:

Laboratory	**3.5-7.2 mg/dL (men)**
	2.6-6.0 mg/dL
	(women)
Nutritional Research	**4.5 – 5.5 mg/dL**

Uric acid is a crystallized acid with the chemical formula $C_5H_4N_4O_3$. Uric acid occurs as an end product of cell metabolism and is normally excreted in the urine. Uric acid is found in the nucleus of kidney and urinary stones (calculi). Uric acid contains a high percentage of ionic nitrogen, which in large concentrations, when not excreted properly can produce exquisite pain, especially in the great toe.

When the blood reading of uric acid is higher than the accepted standard of health, the person most likely consumes large quantities of protein and nitrogenous foods. The uric acid forms crystals that settle in the joints causing a marked increase of pain and calculi in certain parts of the body. Joints become inflamed. Gouty complaints will be prevalent and feature rheumatic conditions, both acute and chronic. Because uric acid is nearly insoluble in water, alcohol, or ether, its remedy forces treatment by certain alkaline salts.

The remedy for high uric acid is to supply the electromagnetic frequencies or substances of: pancreas, kidneys, liver, and thymus; the salts of beryllium, calcium, magnesium, strontium, and barium; bromelain, the amino acids Alanine, aspartic acid, glutamic acid, glycine, vitamin E, folic acid, oat straw, licorice, nettle, skullcap, agrimony, wheat grass juice, blueberries and cherries.

Vegetarian diet, increase fluids.

No alcohol.

When the uric acid reading is lower than the accepted health standard, the person may be on a low protein diet, and certainly may have some symptoms of arthritis, chlorosis (low iron), or possibly heavy metal toxicity. This is a dangerous state of affairs as the toxic buildup of heavy metals (an ever-increasing problem in our modern world) can be most damaging to the body. Lead, cadmium, copper, mercury, and iron severely disrupts the function of the body. These can cause sensory loss, such as blindness, and can ultimately kill a person. A mineral hair analysis should be performed immediately. A low uric acid reading indicates the probability of a blockage or a breakdown in the splitting and cleaving of amino acids, peptides, and polypeptide chains.

The remedy for low uric acid is to supply the electromagnetic frequencies or substances of: pancreatic enzymes (trypsin and chymotrypsin), nucleoproteins, amino acid complex, milk thistle and dandelion leaf.

Heavy metal detoxification formula (Radiation Cocktail—Threat of the Poison Reign), mineral hair analysis.

No coffee.

For customized Energetic, Nutritional Answers:
Go to: www.LifeEnergyResearch.com

- Click "questionnaires." Complete Stress-120 Questionnaire or SAF-120 Questionnaire and receive your chain of numbers.
- Find a Remedy. Access SAFonline and use one or several Interpretations: Juices, Herbs, Homeopathics, Glandulars, Vita Coordinator, Essential Oils, Flower Essences, Chinese Herbs and many more to find the items unique to your chain and your issues.
- Find an SAF practitioner; read about your chain in *SAF Simplified*.

6. Total Cholesterol, serum

Norms:

Laboratory	150-280 mg/100 ml
Nutritional Research	185-215 mg. 100 ml
HDL ("good" cholesterol)	40-85 mg/ 100 ml
LDL ("bad" cholesterol)	100-150 mg/ 100 ml

Cholesterol: the word is derived from the Greek *chole,* which means bile, and *stereos,* which means solid. The chemical configuration is $C_{27}H_{45}OH$, which makes it a fatty alcohol. It is essential for most body tissues, the brain and nervous system, liver and blood. It lubricates the skin and helps with digestion. While cholesterol is an important precursor of adrenal steroid hormones and a vital constituent of many body systems, it remains a controversial subject. The cholesterol reading on a blood chemistry test is the best known.

Cholesterol, being a major plasma lipid, does not circulate freely in solution in the plasma; it is bound to certain complex lipoproteins called chylomicrons. Chylomicrons are:

- very low-density lipoproteins (VLDL)
- low-density lipoproteins (LDL), the "bad" cholesterol because these carry cholesterol to the tissues and deposit them as fat
- High-density lipoproteins (HDL), the "good" cholesterol because these carry cholesterol to the liver for processing and excretion.

Cholesterol is best viewed along with triglycerides to show the exact amount of fatty infiltration in the system. This combination creates the metabolic anomaly of *hyperlipoproteinemia,* which means "high protein-bearing fats in the blood."

When the blood reading for cholesterol is higher than the accepted health standard, it indicates that the body is not handling fats properly. The body may be packing up sterols in the brain, blood, or arteries and advancing the risk of atherosclerosis and hardening of the arteries.

An under active thyroid or obstructive liver disease will raise the level of blood cholesterol. So does the excessive use of alcohol and the action of insulin in diabetics.

The remedy for high cholesterol is to supply the electromagnetic frequencies or substances of: pituitary gland, thyroid, liver; niacin (B3), red rice yeast, essential fatty acids, flax seeds, lecithin, garlic, apples, fenugreek, green tea, Bladderwack, Schisandra, and dandelion.

Low carbohydrate, no alcohol diet, lose weight if necessary.

When the blood reading of cholesterol is lower than the accepted health standard, there is a probability of liver and or gall bladder congestion. As cholesterol originates in the liver and its systems, low blood readings indicate the probability of entrapment. There may be eczema or other skin issues.

The remedy for low cholesterol is to supply the electromagnetic frequencies or substances of: liver, adrenal glands, lecithin, Choline, vitamin E, ginger, milk thistle, raw garlic and onions. Liver detoxification formula.

For customized Energetic, Nutritional Answers:
Go to: www.LifeEnergyResearch.com

- Click "questionnaires." Complete Stress-120 Questionnaire or SAF-120 Questionnaire and receive your chain of numbers.
- Find a Remedy. Access SAFonline and use one or several Interpretations: Juices, Herbs, Homeopathics, Glandulars, Vita Coordinator, Essential Oils, Flower Essences, Chinese Herbs and many more to find the items unique to your chain and your issues.
- Find an SAF practitioner; read about your chain in *SAF Simplified*.

7. Total Protein

Norms:

Laboratory   6.0 – 8.0 g/100 ml
Nutritional Research   7.2 – 7.5 g/100 ml

Protein is the most important component in order for us to help maintain good health, muscle, bones, skin, hair, brain and heart. Protein evaluations reflect the amount of albumin (simple proteins that are water-soluble) and globulins (simple proteins that are not water-soluble) as found in the blood plasma. The anterior pituitary and the gonads, following the growth patterns laid down by the genetic blueprint, coordinate new protein tissue.

When total protein is higher than the accepted health standard, it does not mean the person is eating too much protein but that the protein in the body is being poorly utilized, which might hamper the building of new tissue.

The anterior lobe of the hypophysis (pituitary gland) is responsible for growth hormone production and is often the culprit in hyper protein production.

If the protein level is high, it might indicate infection or inflammation, much mental stress, or it could result from extreme exercise, along with dehydration, that might occur with long distance runners. In the latter case, it will lower soon by itself.

If excessively high it could indicate an underlying disease, which will be addressed by the practitioner.

The remedy for high protein is to supply the electromagnetic frequencies or substances of: the anterior pituitary and the gonads (testes or ovaries), kidneys, trace minerals selenium, manganese, iron, chromium, vanadium and molybdenum (trace amounts found in Bentonite clay), yellow dock, parsley, ginseng, dandelion, and ylang ylang.

Vegetables high in vitamin C will help the kidneys.

When the blood reading of protein is lower than the accepted health standard, there may be a problem of coagulation of protein molecules. There may be poor enzyme action and imperfect cleavage of peptide and polypeptide chains, or bodily stresses such as prolonged illness, surgery, or wounds. There may be lack of vigor, depression or poor resistance to disease.

There may be malnutrition as occurs with digestive disorders. In this case, the food may be nutritious but is not being utilized properly.

The remedy for low protein is to supply the electromagnetic frequencies or substances of: calcium, magnesium, digestive enzymes (protease), St. John's wort, ginseng, and orotic acid (B13). Rich sources of B13 include carrots, beets, and liquid whey.

Increase complete proteins in the diet from organic meat, dairy, eggs or combinations of vegetables and legumes.

For customized Energetic, Nutritional Answers:
Go to: www.LifeEnergyResearch.com
- Click "questionnaires." Complete Stress-120 Questionnaire or SAF-120 Questionnaire and receive your chain of numbers.
- Find a Remedy. Access SAFonline and use one or several Interpretations: Juices, Herbs, Homeopathics, Glandulars, Vita Coordinator, Essential Oils, Flower Essences, Chinese Herbs and many more to find the items unique to your chain and your issues.
- Find an SAF practitioner; read about your chain in *SAF Simplified*.

8. Albumin, serum

Norms:
Laboratory   4.0 – 5.0 g/100 ml
Nutritional Research   4.0 – 4.4 g/100 ml

Albumin is one of the simplest proteins found in the blood serum. It is soluble in cold water and coagulated by heat, after which it is no longer soluble by either hot or cold water. Albumin maintains osmotic pressure in the blood.

Serum albumin acts as a carrier for numerous particles and is involved in plasma osmotic pressure. The amount of serum albumin is determined by its distribution between the intravascular and extravascular areas. It may also be determined by the amount found in the plasma. Although the amount produced by the human liver is as high as 15 grams per day, it is very difficult to use this test as a guideline of liver function because the biological half-life of serum albumin is only 20 days. This places a huge amount of uncertainty upon the reading. It is generally viewed in comparison with globulin readings at the time to dispel any misreading. Many research scientists regard the serum albumin tests as inconclusive, although patients who have chronic liver disease conditions will frequently have decreased amounts of serum albumin.

When the blood reading of albumin is higher than the accepted health standard, there may be a latent condition of arteriosclerosis developing within the blood vessels. This is a problem of the electromagnetic monitoring system of the body (human energy field) being unable to balance the forces within the organism to prevent the excess buildup of the protein in the system. Albumin buildup can occur after overstrain, shock, or when heavy amounts of intolerable stress unleash on the body. The self-protecting system overreacts under stress and reproduces more long chain proteins to send to the sites where the most pressure is felt.

The remedy for high albumin is to supply the electro-magnetic frequencies or substances of: liver, thymus, hypothalamus, orthophosphoric acid, lecithin, chloride, Inositol, Astragalus, thyme, and ginseng.

When the blood reading of albumin is lower than the accepted health standard, there is a chance of kidney disease, liver damage, chronic infection from third degree burns, or intestinal malabsorption. There is the possibility of urinary loss of albumin or a blockage from the buildup of albumin in the liver. Low serum albumin sometimes occurs following weight-loss surgery, Crohn's disease and with low protein diets.

The remedy for low albumin is to supply the electro-magnetic frequencies or substances of: the liver, lecithin, calcium, magnesium, dandelion, cranberry, and aloe.

For customized Energetic, Nutritional Answers:
Go to: www.LifeEnergyResearch.com

- Click "questionnaires." Complete Stress-120 Questionnaire or SAF-120 Questionnaire and receive your chain of numbers.
- Find a Remedy. Access SAFonline and use one or several Interpretations: Juices, Herbs, Homeopathics, Glandulars, Vita Coordinator, Essential Oils, Flower Essences, Chinese Herbs and many more to find the items unique to your chain and your issues.
- Find an SAF practitioner; read about your chain in *SAF Simplified*.

9.   Bilirubin, total

Norms:

Laboratory   .3 – 1.1 mg/100 ml

Nutritional Research   5 – .7 mg/100 ml

Bilirubin is an orange-colored or yellowish pigment in the bile produced by the breakdown of hemoglobin. The bilirubin is an excellent gauge of the infection-fighting capability and the toxin-disposing powers of the body, but the test is used in the lab mainly to discover the possibility of hidden liver disease, such as jaundice.

When the blood reading of total bilirubin is higher than the accepted health standard, it indicates an excessive amount of red blood cells are being destroyed. There is a possibility of an overabundance of liver toxins and the chance that the blood and entire system has been overrun by poison and morbid matter. The bile ducts, which dispose of excess bilirubin into the small intestine, may be blocked or slowed.

Newborns sometimes have elevated bilirubin and special phototherapy (lights) are used to help reduce it.

The remedy for high bilirubin is to supply the electromagnetic frequencies or substances of: the thymus, spleen and bone marrow, iron, vitamins A, vitamin E, B complex vitamins, B1, B5, B6, and B12, milk thistle, burdock, and dandelion.

When the blood reading of the total bilirubin is lower than the accepted health standard, there is a possibility that certain drugs taken to fight infection in the body have decreased the amount of total bilirubin. Drugs such as Phenobarbital (sedative and hypnotic), penicillin and sulfonamides lower the output of bilirubin.

These drugs mentioned interfere with the body's

own anti-infection fighting system. This system produces an electromagnetic web, which is emitted from the brain and the hypothalamus along with the pituitary and the pineal gland (for more information on the human energy field, see *The Origins of Genetic Behavior, The Threat of the Poison Reign,* and *The Promethion* by Joseph R. Scogna, Jr.).

The abuse of any type of antibiotic (which means *anti life*) or infection-fighting over the counter (OTC) medicines will change the protective energy network.

Another cause for reduced bilirubin is an increase in urea backup due to a breakdown or disruption in kidney function.

The remedy for low bilirubin is to supply the electromagnetic frequencies or substances of: the kidney, adrenal glands, pineal, brain, pituitary, bone marrow, spleen, thymus, copper, zinc, phosphorus, vitamin B2, B3, folic acid, garlic, Astragalus, thyme, cranberry, and sage.

For customized Energetic, Nutritional Answers:
Go to: www.LifeEnergyResearch.com
- Click "questionnaires." Complete Stress-120 Questionnaire or SAF-120 Questionnaire and receive your chain of numbers.
- Find a Remedy. Access SAFonline and use one or several Interpretations: Juices, Herbs, Homeopathics, Glandulars, Vita Coordinator, Essential Oils, Flower Essences, Chinese Herbs and many more to find the items unique to your chain and your issues.
- Find an SAF practitioner; read about your chain in *SAF Simplified*.

10. Alkaline Phosphatase (ALP)

Norms:

Laboratory	**20 – 70 IU**
	9.0-35.0 IU

(varies greatly by method)

Nutritional Research   **18.0 – 22.0 IU**

Alkaline Phosphatase (ALP) is an enzyme with the specific function of breaking down the esters of phosphoric acid. These enzymes are extremely important as they convert carbohydrates and phosphorus-bearing fats into energy for the body. They contribute to the formation and metabolism of bone and are found in every tissue of the body. They exist in blood plasma, bone, mammary, spleen, lungs, leukocytes and the adrenal cortex.

The ALP level varies with age. In the first four weeks of life it rises to five or six times the adult norm. After this initial period it drops back slowly until adulthood is reached. Beyond fifty years, there is a slight increase. During the third trimester of pregnancy, alkaline phosphatase may rise to twice its accepted value. After childbirth, it recedes again to normal within two or three weeks after delivery.

When the blood reading of alkaline phosphatase is higher than the accepted health standard, there is the possibility of obstructive jaundice, biliary sclerosis or occlusion of one of the hepatic ducts. There may be lesions in the liver, liver disease, or viral hepatitis. There may be infectious mononucleosis. ALP has been seen to rise with inflammations of the bone, metastatic bone disease, deformities, rickets, and osteomalacia (softening of the bones).

All increases in ALP are evidence of a hypofunction of the adrenal glands, a deteriorating situation in which the adrenal glands fail to spark the ALP conversion process. This weakness of adrenal function causes general debility, dizziness, anxiety and apprehension, and numbness in certain parts of the body.

The remedy for high ALP is to supply the electromagnetic frequencies or substances of: the adrenal glands, hypothalamus, lithium, chloride, sodium, potassium, rubidium, ginseng, and lemon balm.

When the blood reading of alkaline phosphatase is lower than for the accepted health standard, there is the possibility of a hyperfunctioning adrenal gland and a chance the thyroid is also hyperactive. What is taking place in this scenario are the rapid dissolution of alkaline phosphatase and the increased ignition of glucose. Carbohydrate metabolism is markedly disturbed, there may be fleeting but unstable energy. Hypoglycemia may result.

The remedy for low ALP is to supply the electromagnetic frequencies or substances of: the adrenal gland, liver, bone marrow, pancreas, all other glands that may be malfunctioning, B complex vitamins, all the essential amino acids, vitamin C, iodine (kelp), rose hips, horsetail, St. John's Wort, and kava kava.

If hypoglycemic, follow diet on page 17.

For customized Energetic, Nutritional Answers:
Go to: www.LifeEnergyResearch.com

- Click "questionnaires." Complete Stress-120 Questionnaire or SAF-120 Questionnaire and receive your chain of numbers.
- Find a Remedy. Access SAFonline and use one or several Interpretations: Juices, Herbs, Homeopathics, Glandulars, Vita Coordinator, Essential Oils, Flower Essences, Chinese Herbs and many more to find the items unique to your chain and your issues.
- Find an SAF practitioner; read about your chain in *SAF Simplified.*

11. Lactate DeHydrogenase (LDH)
(LDH isoenzymes)

Norms:

Laboratory   **60 – 120 U/ml**
                        95-200 U/ml
(normal ranges vary greatly)

Nutritional Research   80 – 90 U/ml

Lactate Dehydrogenase (LDH) is an enzyme naturally found in several distinct tissues. Its main importance is as a catalyst in the breakdown of lactate in muscle tissue and in other areas of the body. LDH exists in several forms as isoenzymes. Each isoenzyme of LDH relates to a specific tissue area. When tissue is damaged, the specific isoenzymes of LDH for that area (heart, liver, lung, etc.) are released into the blood stream. In this way, certain patterns of LDH can be helpful in determining what tissue area is breaking down.

For example, LDH-1 is associated with the myocardium (heart). This isoenzyme is measured by the amount of electronic flow and speed of the particle in solution. Because it is the most rapidly moving electromagnetic force it was given the title LDH-1.

The slowest moving isoenzyme, LDH-5, originates in the liver. The specific LDH isoenzymes differentiate various conditions such as cardiopulmonary infarction, liver necrosis, and hemolysis. LDH is an intrinsic part of the energy conversion cycle, or Krebs Cycle. These isoenzymes oversee the sugar conversion system of energy and waste products in the tissue. As the tissues make and use energy, these enzymes are called upon to degrade the waste products into water (H_2O) and carbon dioxide (CO_2).

These isoenzymes are needed to make way for new energy.

When the blood reading of LDH is higher than the accepted health standard, there is a condition of blood ionization in various tissues. Depending upon which isoenzymes have been released, there could be problems with the heart or lung areas. An elevated LDH indicates improper balance of energy usage. These enzymes in the blood stream indicate that the body is lagging, energy is low. The metabolic waste products are beginning to build up, not breaking down, as they should. An elevated LDH shows there is an imbalance of sugar usage in all tissues. There may be diabetic symptoms.

The remedy for high LDH is to supply the electromagnetic frequencies or substances of: the pancreas, zinc, chromium, B complex vitamins, niacin (B3), hawthorn berry, and mullein.

If diabetic symptoms, follow diet page 16.

When the blood reading of LDH is lower than the accepted health standard, this may indicate an overuse of glucose in the tissues. Rapid fermentation is occurring and hypoglycemia may exist.

The remedy for low LDH is to supply the electromagnetic frequencies or substances of: the pancreas, folic acid, green tea, chicory, and milk thistle.

Increase complete proteins in the diet; avoid simple carbohydrates (white sugar and flour).

If hypoglycemic, follow diet, page 17.

For customized Energetic, Nutritional Answers:
Go to: www.LifeEnergyResearch.com
- Click "questionnaires." Complete Stress-120 Questionnaire or SAF-120 Questionnaire and receive your chain of numbers.
- Find a remedy. Access SAFonline and use one or several Interpretations: Juices, Herbs, Homeopathics, Glandulars, Vita Coordinator, Essential Oils, Flower Essences, Chinese Herbs and many more to find the items unique to your chain and your issues.
- Find an SAF practitioner; read about your chain in *SAF Simplified*.

12. Asparte Aminotransferase (AST)

(formerly SGOT)

Norms:

Laboratory	**0-41 U/L**
	10 – 40 U/L
(varies greatly by lab)	

Nutritional Research   **18-20 U/L**

Asparte Aminotransferase was formerly called (serum glutamic-oxaloacetic transaminase SGOT). It has been replaced at most labs because AST more closely defines its action.

The enzyme AST is present in many tissues with high metabolic activity. It utilizes glutamic acid and oxaloacetic acid to carry on the process of developing complex compounds for various systems of the body. AST is found in the liver and cardiac regions and is released in the blood stream when either of these systems is injured. As such, it is an extremely valuable guide for measuring cell injury to the hepatic or myocardial area.

When the blood reading of AST is higher than the accepted health standard, there is an increased risk of heart attack and liver disease. Because all tissues possess AST, especially the heart, liver, and skeletal muscles, there is a close relationship between the enzyme and the construction of organ tissue. Glutamic acid is the only amino acid metabolized by the brain and is an important link in the production and hydrolysis of proteins; the anterior pituitary, gonads (testes or ovaries), hypothalamus and thalamus are involved.

If there is a significant increase in AST this may indicate acute liver damage, kidney damage, or metastatic cancer.

In moderate elevations of AST, there may be congestive or enlarged liver, or peripheral muscle disease. There are elevations of AST following consumption of aspirin, cortisone, and codeine. Check for elevated bilirubin because bilirubin has a tendency to momentarily raise AST readings and throw researchers off the track.

The remedy for high AST is to supply the electromagnetic frequencies or substances of: the anterior pituitary, the hypothalamus, B5, B1, and powdered kernels of apricot and apple pits (B17, or Laetrile, also known as amygdalin), hawthorn berry, and essential oil of ylang ylang.

When the reading of AST is lower than the accepted health standard, there is a possibility of malnutrition, hepatic or myocardial tissue blockage. Waste material will cause a slow down in the flow of AST.

The remedy for low AST is to supply the electromagnetic frequencies or substances of: hypothalamus, gonads (testes or ovaries), thymus, spleen, manganese, copper, iron, wheat grass juice, milk thistle, burdock root, white willow bark, and essential oils of rose and ylang ylang, lemon in distilled or reverse osmosis water (Body weight ÷ 2 = # of ounces to drink).

For customized Energetic, Nutritional Answers:
Go to: www.LifeEnergyResearch.com
- Click "questionnaires." Complete Stress-120 Questionnaire or SAF-120 Questionnaire and receive your chain of numbers.
- Find a Remedy. Access SAFonline and use one or several Interpretations: Juices, Herbs, Homeopathics, Glandulars, Vita Coordinator, Essential Oils, Flower Essences, Chinese Herbs and many more to find the items unique to your chain and your issues.
- Find an SAF practitioner; read about your chain in *SAF Simplified*.

13. Total Globulins

Norms:

Laboratory   2.0-3.0 g/100 ml
Nutritional Research   2.5-2.8 g/100 ml

Globulins are simple proteins that are insoluble in pure water but are soluble in saline solutions, strong acids, and strong bases. They help albumin keep water in the blood. There are several globulins in the blood serum of which to take note:

1) Accelerated globulins quicken the conversion of prothrombin to thrombin under the guidance of thromboplastin and calcium ions. This action is essential for blood clotting.

2) Anti-hemophiliac globulin, which is a clotting compound needed for agglutination. This material is deficient in the blood of hemophiliacs.

3) Gamma globulin, which is composed of antibodies to attack viruses, bacterium, and toxins.

4) Alpha and Beta globulins, which are found in blood plasma.

When the blood reading of total globulin is higher than for the accepted health standard, this indicates the presence of unused globulin in the blood stream. This situation often follows a decline of the infection-fighting reticuloendothelial system, and the thyroid, anterior pituitary and hypothalamus. In this case scenario, the coagulation factor and the anti-hemophiliac factors may be present but the organs of the reticuloendothelial system have ceased using globulin to resist viruses, bacteria, and toxins.

Although there may be an acute or chronic presence of these very same invaders and poisons, it is difficult to gauge the effectiveness of the immune system. There may be increased production and use of colloidal protein but this elevated reading would indicate a breakdown in the defense mechanism of the system.

The remedy for high globulin is to supply the electro-magnetic frequencies or substances of: the adrenals, thyroid, thymus, spleen, iron, copper (if copper proves to be deficient by a hair mineral analysis or electromagnetic detection), vitamin C, vitamin A, B2, niacin, super oxide dismutase (SOD), thyme, Astragalus, garlic, green tea, and Bladderwack.

When the blood reading of total globulin is lower than the accepted standard, this would indicate a large number of globulins were being used for repair and fighting infection. There may be a parasitic invasion or the presence of toxins in the system that overwork that globulins.

The remedy for low globulin is to supply the electro-magnetic frequencies or substances of: the thyroid, spleen, thymus glands, calcium, magnesium, phosphorus, folic acid, garlic, silica, oat straw, skullcap, thyme, and cinnamon.

For customized Energetic, Nutritional Answers:
Go to: www.LifeEnergyResearch.com

- Click "questionnaires." Complete Stress-120 Questionnaire or SAF-120 Questionnaire and receive your chain of numbers.
- Find a Remedy. Access SAFonline and use one or several Interpretations: Juices, Herbs, Homeopathics, Glandulars, Vita Coordinator, Essential Oils, Flower Essences, Chinese Herbs and many more to find the items unique to your chain and your issues.
- Find an SAF practitioner; read about your chain in *SAF Simplified*.

14. Albumin/Globulin Ratio (A/G Ratio)

Norms:

Laboratory	**2-4**
Nutritional Research	**2.5-3.5**

The Albumin/Globulin ratio is the image of the blood stream's simple proteins versus the more complex proteins. Albumin and globulin viewed in tandem present an evaluation of the thickness of the blood. The A/G ratio gives the research scientist a good indication as to whether the body is in full-scale reproduction, fighting antibodies, viruses and toxins, or maintaining the normal fibrinogenic texture of the blood.

When the A/G ratio reading is higher than the accepted health standard the blood will be thicker than normal; there will be a persistence of the complex fibrinogen. Fibrinogen is converted into fibrin, which is an integral substance in the process of blood coagulation. The thyroid and the pancreas influence the production of fibrinogen, but the hypothalamus and the thalamus play an even greater role in blood thickness. The acid-alkaline balance of the entire body is dependent upon the correct proportion of protein substances in the blood, and the hypothalamus and thalamus are the main monitors of the blood's hydrogen concentration (pH).

The remedy for high A/G ratio is to supply the electromagnetic frequencies or substances of: the brain, thalamus, pancreas, thymus, spleen, thyroid, hypothalamus, iodine, phosphorus, lemon balm, and yellow dock.

When the A/G ratio is lower than the accepted health standard, the blood in the system shows signs of being too thin. In this scenario, there is a decrease in the presence of complex polypeptide chains and globulins. The clotting factor has been reduced and there is the presence of simple proteins (albumins).

The remedy for low A/G ratio is to supply the electromagnetic frequencies or substances of: the hypothalamus, vitamin K, vitamin E, vitamin A, vitamin D, and lemon balm.

Increase complete proteins to the diet.

For customized Energetic, Nutritional Answers:
Go to: www.LifeEnergyResearch.com

- Click "questionnaires." Complete Stress-120 Questionnaire or SAF-120 Questionnaire and receive your chain of numbers.
- Find a Remedy. Access SAFonline and use one or several Interpretations: Juices, Herbs, Homeopathics, Glandulars, Vita Coordinator, Essential Oils, Flower Essences, Chinese Herbs and many more to find the items unique to your chain and your issues.
- Find an SAF practitioner; read about your chain in *SAF Simplified.*

15. Sodium (Na), serum

Norms:

Laboratory   101-111 m Eq/L or
                              135 – 148 m Eg/l
            (varies by lab)

Nutritional Research   140.0 – 143.0 mEg/l

Sodium (Na+) is a monovalent electrolyte and is principally found in the extra cellular fluids of the body. Its electrical potential in the body governs the balance between calcium and potassium, which regulate heart function and hemostatic equilibrium of the body. Sodium helps to control the amount of intracellular and extracellular H_2O by maintaining electrical balance with potassium and chloride. At this point, the interesting study of electromagnetic principles coordinates directly with blood studies.

The electrical pressure of the elements, particularly sodium, does much to direct and influence the protein substances and enzymes that make up the entire spectrum of blood chemistry. There is little room in this booklet to discuss the vast and intricate network of electrical and electronic influence in the human body (see *The Promethion*). But, it is important to note that sodium is a vital element needed in the function of the adrenal glands, kidneys, bowels, and the fluids of the body.

When the blood reading of sodium is higher than the accepted health standard, there is an indication of stimulated or false acceleration of sodium activity. The pressure of balancing the acid-alkaline relationship of the other elements has become chaotic. The person may experience great dizziness and nervousness, or may be dehydrated or have uremia.

The remedy for high sodium is to supply the electro-magnetic frequencies or substances of: the kidneys, adrenal glands, posterior pituitary, vitamin A, vitamin E, biotin, Choline, B1, B5, B6, B12, all the essential amino acids derived from whole grain, St. John's wort, uva ursi, parsley, dandelion tea, and cucumber juice.

Drink plenty of distilled or reverse osmosis water. (Body weight ÷ 2 = # of ounces to drink).

When the blood reading of sodium is lower than the accepted health standard, this indicates an almost complete usage of sodium ions exclusively in renal function. As a result, the adrenal cortex, along with the posterior pituitary, becomes overworked in the relationship with potassium in trying to maintain osmotic pressure and fluid balance. Potassium may suppress the function of sodium as it vies for union with chloride ions near and in the vicinity of the adrenal glands and the abdominal viscera. This metabolic action usually results in loss of fluids from the body by sweating, copious diarrhea, or frequent urination.

There may be the possibility of undetected diabetes, adrenal insufficiency, or inadequate amounts of antidiuretic hormonal secretions from the posterior pituitary. Diuretics will also decrease the amount of serum sodium levels.

The remedy for low sodium is to supply the electromagnetic frequencies or substances of: adrenal glands, posterior pituitary, sodium in proper balance with potassium, vitamin A, vitamin D, alfalfa, kelp, nettle, red clover, and celery juice.

For customized Energetic, Nutritional Answers:
Go to: www.LifeEnergyResearch.com
- Click "questionnaires." Complete Stress-120 Questionnaire or SAF-120 Questionnaire and receive your chain of numbers.
- Find a Remedy. Access SAFonline and use one or several Interpretations: Juices, Herbs, Homeopathics, Glandulars, Vita Coordinator, Essential Oils, Flower Essences, Chinese Herbs and many more to find the items unique to your chain and your issues.
- Find an SAF practitioner; read about your chain in *SAF Simplified*.

16. Potassium (K), serum

Norms:

Laboratory   2.5-5 m Eq/L
Nutritional Research   3-4 m Eq/L

An essential mineral, potassium is found throughout the intracellular fluids of the body and is necessary for almost every function. It is an electrically charged monovalent cation (positively charged ion) which seeks specific union with chlorides as it duels with sodium for position in the cell membranes. This electrical balance between sodium, potassium, and chloride provides osmotic pressure needed for the implementation of fluid activity, which carries the electric current of the nervous system.

The acid-alkaline balance of the body is dependent upon the movements of sodium and potassium, but more importantly, the specific electrical patterns of potassium form a quadrangle with magnesium, calcium and sodium to maintain electric charge balance and to establish the rhythm of the movements of fluids. A percentage of potassium, which is present in the blood serum, is influenced by any change in pH. The more acid the pH, the more potassium is rejected from the blood serum. The more basic the pH, the more potassium is accepted into the serum.

Potassium helps to keep the skin healthy, stimulates muscle contractions, and converts glucose to glycogen for storage in the liver. Finally, potassium in ionized form works with magnesium to govern the functions of the heart itself.

When the blood reading of potassium is higher than the accepted standard, there is a definite increase in the expulsion of fluid from within the cells, heart action may be labored, and the heart muscle itself must work harder to compensate for the lack of pressure in the cell. Sodium reigns supreme and extracellular fluid increases. Edema will be evident. With a rise in serum levels of potassium there is increased risk of cardiac toxicity. The heart may be overloaded with poisonous wastes. Arteriosclerosis and toxemia, caused by certain digestive disorders and mal-functions of the colon, may present themselves.

The remedy for high potassium is to supply the electro-magnetic frequencies or substances of: the heart, kidney, adrenal glands, vitamin E, vitamin A, the essential fatty acids, flax seed, B1, Pantothenic acid, and evening prim-rose oil.
Increase fiber and drink plenty of fluids.

When the blood reading of potassium is lower than the accepted health standard, there is the possibility that in-tracellular activity has been affected by the use of diuret-ics or certain unbalanced solutions taken to maintain heart pressure. Potassium may be lowered by gastric prob-lems, or intestinal irritations, such as colitis, or if taking cortisone, and there may be the presence of diabetes, renal disease, or adrenal insufficiency. Alcohol and coffee con-sumption cause urinary excretion of potassium.

The remedy for low potassium is to supply the electro-magnetic frequencies or substances of: the pineal, poste-rior pituitary, hypothalamus, niacin, vitamin C, B6, zinc, magnesium, green leafy vegetables, sunflower seeds, mint leaves, potato skins, bananas, and whole grains.
No coffee or alcohol.

For customized Energetic, Nutritional Answers:
Go to: www.LifeEnergyResearch.com
- Click "questionnaires." Complete Stress-120 Questionnaire or SAF-120 Questionnaire and receive your chain of numbers.
- Find a Remedy. Access SAFonline and use one or several Interpreta-tions: Juices, Herbs, Homeopathics, Glandulars, Vita Coordinator, Essential Oils, Flower Essences, Chinese Herbs and many more to find the items unique to your chain and your issues.
- Find an SAF practitioner; read about your chain in *SAF Simplified*.

17. Chloride (Cl), serum

Norms:

Laboratory   98-106 m Eq/L
Nutritional Research 102-104 m Eq/L

Chloride is a negatively charged anion, monovalent in nature. The element combines with sodium in the blood to exert influence over the osmotic pressure between cell activity as it relates to tissue and organ function, at the same time avoiding electrical pressure from potassium. Chloride aids in digestion, stimulates gastric enzymes and is a primary metabolic element in the oxidation of proteins, albumin, and globulins in solution. Chloride is stored in the medulla of the adrenal gland and transmits its power through almost every cell in the body with the assistance of the hypothalamus.

When the blood reading of chloride is higher than the accepted health standard, it may indicate a trauma, accident, chronic illness, diabetes, or other hidden undetected ailments of long duration. Chloride, in coordination with the hypothalamus, posterior pituitary, adrenal glands and the kidneys, work to expel used fluids and byproducts of energy usage (carbon dioxide & water) out through the urinary system. High blood readings indicate possible bowel and bladder malfunctions involving the kidneys and adrenal glands.

The remedy for high chloride is to supply the electromagnetic frequencies or substances of: hypothalamus, posterior pituitary, adrenals, kidneys, stomach or intestinal substances, HCl, potassium, with orotic acid (B13), essential fatty acids, flax seed, evening primrose oil, cranberry, carrots, beets, and liquid whey.

When the blood reading of chloride is lower than the accepted health standard, this may indicate that chloride is trapped in insoluble salts in the body and can only be brought up to its normal stable reading by degradation of new hydrogen ionization. This degradation will have to come by way of the electromagnetic commands of the hypothalamus, in coordination with the adrenal glands.

There may be hair and tooth loss, and poor digestion.

The remedy for low chloride is to supply the electromagnetic frequencies or substances of: the hypothalamus, adrenal glands, tissue salt of sodium chloride (natrum muriaticum), silica, ginseng, B2, B3, vitamin C, chamomile, ginger, sarsaparilla, and lemon balm.

For customized Energetic, Nutritional Answers:
Go to: www.LifeEnergyResearch.com
- Click "questionnaires." Complete Stress-120 Questionnaire or SAF-120 Questionnaire and receive your chain of numbers.
- Find a Remedy. Access SAFonline and use one or several Interpretations: Juices, Herbs, Homeopathics, Glandulars, Vita Coordinator, Essential Oils, Flower Essences, Chinese Herbs and many more to find the items unique to your chain and your issues.
- Find an SAF practitioner; read about your chain in *SAF Simplified.*

18. Carbon Dioxide (CO₂), serum

Norms:
Laboratory   23-30 mmol/L
Nutritional Research   21-25 mmol/L

Carbon dioxide (CO_2) is an odorless gas. It results from the explosion of carbon and oxygen as it is being used for energy in the body so it is useful to evaluate the acid-alkaline balance. Carbon dioxide is essential as a compound of the Krebs Cycle of Energy Conversion (Tricarboxylic acid cycle) which demonstrates the methodical chain reactions of sugars, fatty acids, and proteins to produce carbon dioxide, water and high-energy phosphate bonds that are used for energy and action.

Carbon dioxide is eliminated through every available channel of the body; its loss is directly related to glucose usage in every cell and tissue of the body. There is a constant push-pull within the body, with homeostasis or balance the result. In the lungs, an abundance of carbon dioxide instigates the respiration of oxygen and so, by monitoring the CO_2 levels in blood serum, a correlation can be drawn regarding lung capacity as well. If found in great quantities, carbon dioxide can produce mental confusion, irregular breathing, and death by suffocation.

Carbon dioxide blood testing is monitored to determine the amount of the compound that can be held by the blood serum. The person's blood is merely breathed upon, then measured. This reading gives researchers an idea of how much CO_2 the blood can hold before exploding in its crave for oxygen.

When the blood reading for carbon dioxide is higher than the accepted health standard, there is the possibility of lung congestion. In this case, the tissues are unable to expel the products of combustion properly and CO_2 spills hectically into the blood stream. There may be vomiting and pulmonary disease.

The remedy for high carbon dioxide is to supply the electromagnetic frequencies or substances of: the lungs, vitamin A, magnesium, sulfur-bearing amino acids containing Methionine and lysine, ginger, peppermint, lemon balm, elderberry, and elecampane.

When the blood reading for carbon dioxide is lower than the accepted health standard, there is a chance that the lungs have lost some capacity for exhalation and inhalation. This is the direct responsibility of the organism's genetic strength factor, emitting from the thalamus and the brain, monitoring cardiopulmonary function. The adrenal glands and the thyroid play important roles in metering the volume of air that is allowed in proportion to what can be converted to carbon dioxide. This is the scenario of a person who may develop weak lungs. It may be low from diabetes, kidney disease or hyperventilation.

The remedy for low carbon dioxide is to supply the electromagnetic frequencies or substances of: the lung, adrenal glands, heart, hypothalamus, thalamus, brain, thyroid, lemon balm, barberry, hawthorn berry, Flavonoid rich foods, yarrow, and ginkgo.

For customized Energetic, Nutritional Answers:
Go to: www.LifeEnergyResearch.com
- Click "questionnaires." Complete Stress-120 Questionnaire or SAF-120 Questionnaire and receive your chain of numbers.
- Find a Remedy. Access SAFonline and use one or several Interpretations: Juices, Herbs, Homeopathics, Glandulars, Vita Coordinator, Essential Oils, Flower Essences, Chinese Herbs and many more to find the items unique to your chain and your issues.
- Find an SAF practitioner; read about your chain in *SAF Simplified*.

19. Creatinine ($C_4H_7ON_3$), serum

Creatinine means *flesh* in Greek. It is the end product of the metabolism of creatinine phosphate, which is a high-energy substance created in muscle tissue. It is therefore a significant substance in the rebuilding tissues and in the generation and evolution of <u>action</u> for the organism. This action involves the combustion of glucosides (sugars) to produce muscle contractions. Therefore, blood evaluation of creatinine is an excellent gauge of muscle contraction. Elevated levels of creatinine have been found in advanced stages of kidney disease and are one of the best monitors to detect early stage renal damage.

When the creatinine reading is higher than the accepted health standard, there is evidence of faltering muscle action as the creatinine phosphate is being inefficiently converted into creatinine at a higher rate than normal. An elevated level of creatinine suggests a possibility of muscle tissue breakdown as can be seen with weightlifters. The creatinine levels increase significantly with a severe workout and the level decreases with a less severe workout.

The remedy for a high creatinine is to supply the electromagnetic frequencies or substances of: the anterior pituitary, gonads, adrenal glands, vitamin E, vitamin A, B15 (calcium pangamate), and orotic acid (B13), carrot and beet juice, and liquid whey.

When the blood reading of creatinine is lower than the accepted health standard, there is the risk of muscle wasting or atrophy. In this case, not enough creatinine is produced because of the snarls and blockages in muscle tissues created by the sclerosis of hemoglobin in the muscle.

The remedy for low creatinine is to supply the electromagnetic frequencies or substances of: the pituitary, thyroid, parathyroid, adrenal glands, pineal, gonads, pancreas, B6, lecithin, vitamin E, and hydrochloric acid (HCl) if not allergic.

Increase complete proteins in the diet.

For customized Energetic, Nutritional Answers:
Go to: www.LifeEnergyResearch.com

- Click "questionnaires." Complete Stress-120 Questionnaire or SAF-120 Questionnaire and receive your chain of numbers.
- Find a Remedy. Access SAFonline and use one or several Interpretations: Juices, Herbs, Homeopathics, Glandulars, Vita Coordinator, Essential Oils, Flower Essences, Chinese Herbs and many more to find the items unique to your chain and your issues.
- Find an SAF practitioner; read about your chain in *SAF Simplified*.

20. Iron (Fe), serum

Norms:

Laboratory	**75-175 mcg/100 ml men**
	65-165 mcg/100 ml women
Nutritional Research	**95-100 mcg/100 ml**

There is one fact indisputable in all scientific ledgers - iron is essential to life!

This element, when combined with protein and copper, plays an important role in the formation of hemoglobin to combat anemia. Hemoglobin transports oxygen to the cells and tissues; without it, there would be no carrier for oxygen. The transmission of the carbon cycle of existence would cease – the organism would die. Iron participates with enzymes in cellular respiration and in the energy creation cycle.

When the blood reading of iron is higher than the accepted health standard, the immediate probability is an electronic breakdown in a system caused by insulation that has jammed the transmission of oxygen. Excess fats and oils in the blood stream cause this type of breakdown. Those who consume large amounts of saturated and unsaturated fats will inadvertently block the corridors that use iron to carry its payload of oxygen, thereby suppressing the valuable function of energy creation. There could be genetic factors, blood transfusions or a high intake of iron.

The remedy for high iron is to supply the electromagnetic frequencies or substances of: the thymus, spleen, liver, B12, Bentonite clay (colloidal suspension), B3 (niacin), lipase (made from pancreatic substance), lecithin, B6, and apple cider vinegar.

When the blood reading of iron is lower than the accepted health standard, there is a risk of iron deficiency anemia.

The remedy for low iron is to supply the electromagnetic frequencies or substances of: liver, thymus, adrenal glands, spleen, iron, the left side nutrients manganese, chromium, molybdenum, and vanadium as found in Bentonite clay, folic acid, molasses, dandelion salad, parsley, iron rich foods (organic liver, heart), green leafy vegetables, asparagus, and organic and inorganic iron salts.

For customized Energetic, Nutritional Answers:
Go to: www.LifeEnergyResearch.com
- Click "questionnaires." Complete Stress-120 Questionnaire or SAF-120 Questionnaire and receive your chain of numbers.
- Find a Remedy. Access SAFonline and use one or several Interpretations: Juices, Herbs, Homeopathics, Glandulars, Vita Coordinator, Essential Oils, Flower Essences, Chinese Herbs and many more to find the items unique to your chain and your issues.
- Find an SAF practitioner; read about your chain in *SAF Simplified*.

21. BUN/Creatinine Ratio

Norms:

Laboratory	11-24
Nutritional Research	14.5-15.5

Creatinine is a result of the breakdown of muscle metabolism and is excreted into the urine. Therefore, this substance found in blood serum can be a good measure of renal function.

Creatinine is not as sensitive as the blood urea nitrogen (BUN) in reading the early stages of kidney damage and so must be compared with the BUN reading for that purpose. The BUN is much more precise and helps to differentiate what area of the kidney is under the most stress. The main "search and discovery" is targeted to find the location of nitrogenous wastes in the system along with the imbalance of H_2O, glucose, carbon dioxide, and the essential trace elements.

When the blood reading of the BUN/Creatinine ratio is higher than the accepted health standard, it indicates repeated fluid loss somewhere in the system and the possibility of pre-renal or post-renal obstructions of nitrogenous wastes (ammonia, nitrates, nitrites, etc.). This is an early sign of kidney damage, and or pituitary malfunction. With the loss of minerals, the electric charge capability has been reduced.

The remedy for high BUN/Creatinine ratio is to supply the electromagnetic frequencies or substances of: the posterior pituitary, kidneys, adrenals, a multi-mineral complex, calcium carbonate, red clover, raspberry, alfalfa, nettle, and carrot juice.

Drink plenty of distilled or reverse osmosis water.

When the blood reading of BUN/Creatinine is lower than the accepted health standard, there is the inverse problem of an increase of fluids in the system, which may back up and cause swelling of tissues in the entire body. Again there is the possibility of nitrogenous wastes backing up within the blood stream and the breakdown of healthy tissue.

The remedy for low BUN/Creatinine is to supply the electromagnetic frequencies or substances of: the posterior pituitary, kidneys, calcium orotate, calcium pangamate, Proteolytic enzymes, dandelion, parsley and cucumber juice.

For customized Energetic, Nutritional Answers:
Go to: www.LifeEnergyResearch.com
- Click "questionnaires." Complete Stress-120 Questionnaire or SAF-120 Questionnaire and receive your chain of numbers.
- Find a Remedy. Access SAFonline and use one or several Interpretations: Juices, Herbs, Homeopathics, Glandulars, Vita Coordinator, Essential Oils, Flower Essences, Chinese Herbs and many more to find the items unique to your chain and your issues.
- Find an SAF practitioner; read about your chain in *SAF Simplified*.

---

22. Triglycerides, serum

Norms:

| Laboratory | 40-160 mg/100 ml men |
| | 35-135 mg/100 ml women |

Nutritional Research   95-105 mg/100 ml

A triglyceride is a compound of several molecules of fatty acids and glycerol. Blood serum levels indicate the body's ability to metabolize fats. Fatty acids are synthesized from carbohydrates and then stored in the adipose (fat) tissues of animals. Triglyceride readings are generally observed in tandem with cholesterol and when elevated indicate a condition of *hyperlipidemia* (high protein bearing fats in the blood). As stated in Section 6 (Cholesterol) these fats are transported in macromolecular complexes of lipoproteins called chylomicrons. Chylomicrons are:

- very low-density lipoproteins (VLDL)
- low-density lipoproteins (LDL), the "bad" cholesterol because they carry cholesterol to the tissues and deposit them as fat
- High-density lipoproteins (HDL), the "good" cholesterol because they carry cholesterol to the liver for processing and excretion.

When compared with cholesterol and any phospholipid, triglycerides are the major portion of fats transported through the blood. The main source of an elevated triglyceride is the interruption of the rhythm of electromagnetic energy around the body, which then creates fatty deposits for insulation and protection. This action is a means of buffering high intensity stress, trauma, shock, toxins, poisons, bacteria, and viruses.

When both cholesterol and triglyceride levels are elevated, it indicates a high risk of atherosclerosis (fat buildup or hardening of the arteries). Other chemistry findings may include pancreatitis, enlarged spleen, enlarged liver, eruptive xanthomas (yellowish tumors), glucose intolerance, and high serum uric acid.

When the blood reading of triglycerides is higher than the accepted health standard, it shows that fatty acids are not being used properly by the nervous system to correct and block the excesses of electric charge in the system. Therefore the fats, complexed with glycerol, are beginning to buildup and overcompensate to alleviate traumas, stress, pain, shock, and injury.

It is interesting to note that the trauma may have long since passed, but the body, in an endless attempt to correct the old situation, continues to build up insulation in the form of triglycerides. The remedy is to first remove the main source and cause of disturbance toward the body. This may be stress, systemic toxins or poisons, such as lead or other metals, or allergic substances.

Lowering the consumption of fatty meats will help to reduce fat deposits and weight in the entire system, but it is essential to reduce or remove the stresses generated from outside the body (exogenous) and stress generated from inside the body (endogenous). The electric pressure of stress keeps the cells, the tissues, and the organs and glands in a non-fluid state of constant aggravation.

The SAF Stress – 120 Questionnaire is a holistic health evaluation that can point to the emotional issues that may be causing stress as well as present a priority order. (www.LifeEnergyResearch.com Stress Questionnaire, then seek an SAF practitioner for interpretation).

A detoxification program will help to flush out systemic toxins found in the Radiation Cocktail and Detox Program, in *The Threat of the Poison Reign* by Joseph R. Scogna, Jr.

For allergies, determine and remove from diet, home or environment those substances that aggravate and overwhelm. Use the SAFonline interpretations Remedy Orange, Millennium Detox, and use homeopathic remedies.

(See also *The Origins of Genetic Behavior*.)

The remedy for high triglycerides is to supply the electromagnetic frequencies or substances of: the hypothalamus, pituitary, and pancreas, vitamin C, B3 (niacin), fat-splitting enzymes, raw garlic and onions, milk thistle, yellow dock, burdock root, ginseng, fenugreek, valerian, and lemon balm.

Identify and remove sources of stress and disturbance. (Stress 120 Questionnaire, then Emotion Hazards.)

Detoxify the liver; reduce the amount of fatty meats consumed; increase distilled or reverse-osmosis water consumption (Body weight ÷ 2 = # of ounces to drink)

Non-invasive allergy testing (Remedy Orange, Millennium Detox at SAFonline).

Exercise more (walking, biking, gym workouts as tolerated).

When the blood reading for triglycerides is lower than the accepted health standard, there may be a jam-up between fat-producing hormones and the energy field, which maintains harmony within the body as well as without. There may be a condition of overwhelm in the system, caused by physical, mental or spiritual stressors, that is intensified without the buffering effect of triglycerides.

The remedy for low triglycerides is to supply the electromagnetic frequencies or substances of: liver, pineal gland, lecithin, Choline, raw garlic and onions, ginseng, milk thistle, Astragalus, and thyme.

For customized Energetic, Nutritional Answers:
Go to: www.LifeEnergyResearch.com

- Click "questionnaires." Complete Stress-120 Questionnaire or SAF-120 Questionnaire and receive your chain of numbers.
- Find a Remedy. Access SAFonline and use one or several Interpretations: Juices, Herbs, Homeopathics, Glandulars, Vita Coordinator, Essential Oils, Flower Essences, Chinese Herbs and many more to find the items unique to your chain and your issues.
- Find an SAF practitioner; read about your chain in *SAF Simplified*.

23. Alanine Aminotransferase (ALT)
(formerly SGPT)

Norms:

Laboratory	**7-24 U/L men**
	7-17 U/L women
Nutritional Research	**18-22 U/L**

Alanine Aminotransferase (ALT) was formerly called SGPT (serum glutamic-pyruvic transaminase). It has been replaced at most labs because ALT more closely defines its function

Alanine Aminotransferase (ALT) catalyzes the conversion of Alanine and ketoglutaric acid (part of the Krebs Cycle of Energy Conversion) to produce pyruvic and glutamic acids respectively. The ALT reading is similar to the AST mentioned previously. Both are vital to energy production in the body and are released into the blood stream whenever specific tissues are damaged. ALT is released in liver damage whereas AST is released during injury or breakdown of the heart muscle.

The ALT enzyme is closely associated with the conversion of glucose ($C_2H_{12}O_6$), oxygen and carbon dioxide. The function of the adrenal glands, lungs, liver, kidneys, and pituitary gland is also influenced by ALT. ALT is essential in the lifeline of vital organs and when injured, indicate imbalance with one another.

When the blood reading of ALT is higher than the accepted health standard, there is a chance of a multitude of tissue breakdown or damage and disturbance in the energy conversion cycle. There may be frontal headaches, sinus pain, or a coated tongue.

The remedy for high ALT is to supply the electromagnetic frequencies or substances of: liver, kidneys, adrenals, vitamin E, B complex vitamins, milk thistle, dandelion, cranberry, and ginseng.

When the blood reading of ALT is lower than the accepted health standard, there is a risk of damage to the liver tissue so severe that production of the necessary enzymes may be halted altogether or very nearly so.

The remedy for low ALT is to supply the electromagnetic frequencies or substances of: liver, pituitary, iron, niacin, alfalfa, raspberry, nettle, and yellow dock.

For customized Energetic, Nutritional Answers:
Go to: www.LifeEnergyResearch.com

- Click "questionnaires." Complete Stress-120 Questionnaire or SAF-120 Questionnaire and receive your chain of numbers.
- Find a Remedy. Access SAFonline and use one or several Interpretations: Juices, Herbs, Homeopathics, Glandulars, Vita Coordinator, Essential Oils, Flower Essences, Chinese Herbs and many more to find the items unique to your chain and your issues.
- Find an SAF practitioner; read about your chain in *SAF Simplified*.

24. Thyroxine (T$_4$)

Norms:

Laboratory	4.4-9.9 mcg/100 ml
	5-12.5 mcg/100 ml

(varies greatly by lab)

Nutritional Research 6.5-7 mcg/100 ml

Thyroxine is an iodine-containing hormone secreted by the thyroid gland, whose purpose is to regulate the rate of cell metabolism. The T$_4$ (tetraiodothyronine or thyroxine) test measures thyroid function. It is accomplished by exposing a patient's T$_4$ to thyroxine-binding globulin (TGB) immersed in radioactive iodine T$_4$. A balance in lateral readings takes place between the radioactive T$_4$ and the patient's T$_4$. These two measurements are compared and the reading is rendered.

The basis of this test is centered on the protein-bound iodine (PBI). The element iodine binds up with colloidal proteins of the thyroid gland to carry out specific metabolic functions including stabilizing oxygen, carbon dioxide and maintaining homeostasis of the carbon-nitrogen cycles. This makes iodine "lord of the realm" when it comes to resisting infection and in working with the thyroid, thymus, and spleen.

When the blood value of T$_4$ is higher than the accepted health standard, this may indicate hyperthyroidism, or overactive thyroid. The body is beginning to step up its conversion process and as a result more waste products accumulate in the body. The system begins to vacillate toward the nitrogen side of the cycle.

Elevated thyroid may be caused by heredity or emotional stress and can lead to irritability, fatigue, goiter and rapid pulse.

57

The remedy for high thyroid is to supply the electro-magnetic frequencies or substances of: thyroid, liver, anterior pituitary, iodine (kelp), sulfur-bearing amino acids lysine and Methionine, B vitamins, kava kava, valerian, horsetail, and St. John's wort.
Determine the emotional stressors
Detoxification program is needed.

When the blood reading of T_4 is lower than the accepted health standard, this may indicate hypothyroid, or a low functioning thyroid gland. This scenario indicates a slowdown in the conversion of oxygen to carbon dioxide and the body is vibrating toward the carbon side of the cycle. There may be a gain in weight toward obesity, myxedema, and metabolic disorders associated with a sluggish thyroid. There may be emotional issues. The SAF Stress-120 Questionnaire is a holistic health evaluation that can point to the emotional issues that may be causing stress, as well as present a priority order.

The remedy for low thyroid is to supply the electromagnetic frequencies or substances of: the thyroid, spleen, thymus, vitamin B complex, vitamin A, vitamin C, calcium, Inositol, carrot juice, green tea, basil essential oil, and an herb tincture of Schisandra berry, nettle, dandelion leaf, Guggel, ginseng, and Bladderwack.
Discover and address emotional stressors.
Increase fiber. Add complete proteins to the diet.
Avoid coffee, tea, nicotine, and alcohol.

For customized Energetic, Nutritional Answers:
Go to: www.LifeEnergyResearch.com

- Click "questionnaires." Complete Stress-120 Questionnaire or SAF-120 Questionnaire and receive your chain of numbers.
- Find a Remedy. Access SAFonline and use one or several Interpretations: Juices, Herbs, Homeopathics, Glandulars, Vita Coordinator, Essential Oils, Flower Essences, Chinese Herbs and many more to find the items unique to your chain and your issues.
- Find an SAF practitioner; read about your chain in *SAF Simplified*.

25. Complete Blood Count (CBC)

Nutritional Research Norms:

RBC	4.5 – 5 million / uL men
	3.6—5 million /uL women
WBC	5,000 –10,000 / uL
Lymphocytes	20% - 35% of all WBCs
Neutrophils	50% - 60% of granulocytes
Eosinophils	0% - 2% of granulocytes
Basophils	0% - 2% of granulocytes
Monocytes	0% - 2% of all WBCs

The blood serum is actually classified as connective tissue. Blood is composed of red blood cells (RBCs), white blood cells (WBCs), and plasma, the colorless, liquid portion. It is pumped by the heart and transported by way of arteries, veins, and capillaries. Its most important purpose is to transport oxygen and essential nutrients to the cells and tissues of the body. After the cycle of energy and the transactions of enzymes are completed, the carbon dioxide and other metabolic wastes are removed from the sites and transported to certain organs for disposal.

The Complete Blood Count (CBC) is used as a basic screening to detect anemia, inflammations, and leukemia. Drugs, medicines and their side effects are also investigated. In the standard CBC a determination is made of the hemoglobin, hematocrit, white blood count, and red blood count (including size and shape). The plasma (colorless fluid of the blood) contains various vital substances and different types of cells.

Red Blood Cells (RBC)

The red blood cells or erythrocytes (RBC) are the most abundant, numbering between 3 and 5 million per cubic millimeter of blood. The RBCs have a life-sustaining role, as it is with the RBCs that the prolific exchange of life energy between the environment (oxygen) and the organism (carbon) is made. To successfully carry out this exchange, the RBCs must have the proper quota of hemoglobin (iron and protein) and oxygen. Its red pigment is proportionate to the amount of iron that it carries; the more oxygen, the brighter red the color.

Anemia, a condition of low iron, means *lack of blood*. Without iron, there is a lack of blood; without blood there is a lack of the necessary creations and reactions of life energy.

RBCs originate as young nuclei in the bone marrow and as they come of age they lose their nucleus, form into a disc and then begin to manufacture hemoglobin. The life of the red blood cell is about 120 days, after which the spleen destroys them. The system of grouping individuals by blood type, such as O, A, B, AB, Rh- and Rh+ comes directly from the differences of structure on and around the cells, which vary from person to person.

When the blood count of the RBC is higher than the accepted health standard, this may indicate a very large capacity for carrying oxygen and nutrients to each cell site, but there could dehydration, or polycythemia as occurs at a high altitude. There may be a breakdown of splenic function; the spleen is the RBCs final destination and it is possible not enough RBCs are being destroyed.

To remedy or stabilize any imbalance in the RBC value (high or low), provide the electromagnetic frequencies of: the spleen, adrenal, hypothalamus, thyroid, and kidneys.

When the blood chemistry indicates the RBC is low, increase the protein intake and iron-rich foods such as organic meat, parsley, dandelion root, ginkgo, molasses, and raw bone concentrates.

White Blood Cells (WBC)

The leukocytes (white blood cells or WBCs) are programmed to defend the body on all fronts against infections and the invasions of alien microorganisms, bacteria, and viruses. The WBCs carry on this action everywhere in the body, including within the blood stream.

But sometimes, in their zeal to protect the body, the WBC run amuck and multiply in great numbers. When they increase well beyond their normal 5,000 to 10,000 per cubic milliliter of blood, this may indicate leukemia. Because WBCs also increase significantly in the presence of infection, it is believed that a virus with which the body cannot cope may cause leukemia. In this scenario, the WBCs continue to reproduce in high numbers and then are ineffective to fight infection, which was their original purpose.

On the other hand, a low number of WBCs indicates lowered resistance, and an increased chance of infection and invasion by unwanted parasites and the like.

The destruction of WBCs occurs usually from the overuse and abuse of drugs and medicines of all kinds. WBCs circulate in the blood only about 6-8 hours, but then enter body tissues and live longer.

When the WBC in general is higher than the accepted health standard, there may be an overwhelming infection in the body. This infection may be taxing the immune system, which needs immediate assistance to destroy the invaders, as well as rid the body of other toxic waste. There also could be dehydration.

The remedy of high WBC is to supply the electromagnetic frequencies or substances of: the hypothalamus, spleen, thymus, and liver.

Detoxification formula to include high doses of vitamin A, vitamin C, vitamin E, zinc, garlic and lemon balm.

Increase distilled or reverse osmosis water intake.

When the WBC is lower than the accepted health standard, there is the basis for the belief that excess toxicity pervades the system with bone marrow suppression.

The remedy for a low WBC is to provide the electromagnetic frequencies or substances of: thymus gland, liver, bone marrow, dandelion, vitamins A, C, E, zinc, iron, Bioflavonoids, boneset, Echinacea, and Astragalus.

A liver detoxification program is needed.

There are three types of leucocytes (WBCs).

1) Granulocytes – These WBC cells are divided into three groups:

The neutrophils, segmented and immature, are neutral in the presence of acid or alkaline dye. They are programmed to attack and destroy by enveloping any bacteria or microorganisms that may be harmful to the body.

Neutrophils: When the neutrophils become unstable, either high or low, supply the electromagnetic frequencies or substance of: the spleen and the thymus glands.

The eosinophils, which react very positively to alkaline dyes, comprise 1-3% of the granulocytes. Its action and increase is triggered by the presence of allergic substances and parasites that may infest the gut membrane of the body.

The basophils, which react very positively to alkaline dyes, comprise less than 1% of the total granulocytes. Their main action is to assist in defending against parasites, allergies, inflammatory reactions, and in balancing the blood clot mechanism of the body. As mast cells, basophils reside along blood vessels.

Eosinophils & basophils. Supply the electromagnetic frequency or substance of: pancreatic enzymes, hydrochloric acid (HCl), barberry, thyme, and garlic.

2) Lymphocytes- These comprise 20-40% of all the WBCs. The lymphocytes do most of their immunity work in the plasma by producing forces of repulsion against microorganisms: T-cells are thymus-derived; B cells produce anti-bodies; natural killer cells (NK) are found in spleen, bone marrow, blood and lymph nodes.

When the lymphocytes vacillate away from the norm, there is a definite major disturbance in the defense system of the body. If high, it may be a viral infection. If low, there is dangerous susceptibility to infection.

Lymphocytes: the remedy for changes would be to supply the electromagnetic frequency or substances of: the spleen and thymus, silica, garlic, and cleansing herbs milk thistle, cleavers, rosemary, and sarsaparilla.

3) Monocytes- These WBC cells connect into a vast network of defense called the reticuloendothelial system. The monocytes are generally the "clean-up crew" when it comes to the ravages of war waged by the other WBC cells against the invaders in the body. In other words the monocytes phagocytize the debris left by other WBCs. In this way, their elevated number is a very good gauge of just how rapidly tissue is breaking down and how much specific infection there may be. As macrophages, these reside in the liver, spleen and lymph nodes.

It is in the chronic diseases, such as pneumonia, typhoid, and malaria where the monocytes do most of their work.

Monocytes: When the monocytes are higher than the accepted health standard, supply the electromagnetic frequency or substance of: liver, spleen, thymus, vitamin E, selenium, B12, garlic, thyme, barberry, Pau d'arco, and primary anti-oxidants vitamin C and vitamin A.

References & Further Reading:

Bagnell: Clinical Procedures, 1979

Boericke: *Homeopathic Materia Medica*, 9th Edition, Boericke & Runyon, Philadelphia 1927

Dorland's Illustrated Medical Dictionary – 28th Edition, W. B. Saunders, 1974

Harrar-O'Donnell, *The Woman's Book of Healing Herbs*, Rodale Press, 1999

I-San Lin, Dr. Robert: *Garlic and Health*, International Academy of Health and Fitness, Inc. 1994

Massachusetts General Hospital Laboratory Values for SMAC-24

Memmler, Cohan, Wood: *The Human Body in Health and Disease*, Lippincott, 1996

Merck Manual – 13th Edition, Merck and Co., Inc. 1977

Micro-Dyn: *Materia Medica (homeopathic)*, Northwest Botanicals, Sumas, Washington, 1978

Miller-Keane, *Encyclopedia and Dictionary of Medicine, Nursing and Allied Health*, WB Saunders, CO., 1983

Page, Jake: *Blood: The River of Life*, U.S. News Books. 1981

Reader's Digest, *Magic and Medicine of Plants*, 1989

Russian Experimental Findings of Pangamate of Calcium, Vitamin B15, its Efficacy and Uses in the Treatment of Heart Disease, 1978

SAFonline Questionnaires & Remedy Interpretations LifeEnergyResearch.com, SAFonline: 1980 - 2014 (Herbs, Homeopathics, Remedy Orange, Juice, Essential Oils, Mood, Remedy Red, Vita Coordinator, Chinese Herbs, etc.)

Scogna, Joseph R. Jr.: *The Blood Works*, Life Energy Publications, 1980

Scogna, Joseph R., Jr. & Kathy M. Scogna: *The Homeopathic Self-Appraisal Index,* Life Energy Publications, 2005

Scogna, Joseph R., Jr. & Kathy M. Scogna: *The Origins of Genetic Behavior: the Handbook for Human Healing,* 2014

Scogna, Joseph R. Jr.: *The Promethion*, Life Energy Publications, 1980, (2003 Kathy M. Scogna, Editor)

Scogna, Joseph R. Scogna, Jr.: *The Threat of the Poison Reign*, Life Energy Publications, 1980, (2005 Kathy M. Scogna, Editor)

Scogna, Kathy M.: *Amino Acids: A Nutritional Guide*, Life Energy Publications, 1983, 2005

Scogna, Kathy M. editor, compiler, *SAF Simplified*, Life Energy Publications, 2003

Index

Adrenal Glands,13, 16, 17, 21, 27, 29, 35, 39, 41, 42, 43,45,46,47,49,50,56,60
Agrimony, 18
Alanine, 18
Alanine Aminotransferase, (ALT) (formerly SGPT), 55-56
Albumin, serum 24-25
Albumin/Globulin (A/G) Ratio,36-37
Alcohol, 18,21,41,58
Alfalfa,9,39,50,56
Alkaline Phosphatase 28-29
Allergies,62
Allergy Testing, 54
Aloe, 25
Amino Acids,19,29,39
Ammonium Chloride, 12
Amygdalin,33
Amylase,10
Anterior Pituitary,17,22,33,46,58
Apple cider vinegar, 48
Apple pits, powdered,33
Apples, 16,17,21Apricot kernels, powdered, 33
Artificial ingredients/sweeteners, 17
Asparagus, 49
Asparte Aminotransferase (AST)(formerly SGOT), 32-33
Aspartic Acid, 18
Astragalus, 24,27,35,54,62

Bananas,41
Barberry, 45,62,63
Barium, homeopathic, 17,25
Barium, salt, 18
Basil, essential oil, 58
Beets, 23,42
Beet Juice, 46
Bentonite clay, 48,49
Beryllium, salt, 18
Bilirubin, Total, 26-27
Bioflavonoids, 62
Biotin 39
Bladderwack, 21, 35,58
Blood Urea Nitrogen (BUN), 13-14
Blueberries, 18

Blueberry Leaf tea, 16
Bone Marrow, 26,27,29,62
Bone Set, 62
Brain,16,17,27,36,45
Bromelain, 18
BUN/Creatinine Ratio, 50-51
Burdock Root, 26,33,54

Calcium (Ca), 9-10, 17, 23, 25, 35, 58
Calcium Carbonate, 50
Calcium Orotate, 51
Calcium Pangamate, 46, 51
Calcium, ionized, 10
Calcium, salt, 18
Chamomile, 9,43
Carbon Dioxide (CO_2), serum, 44-45
Carrots,23,42
Carrot Juice,10,46,50,58
Celery Juice, 39
Cherries, 18
Chicory, 31
Chloride (Cl), 25,29,42-43
Cholesterol, Total, serum, 20-21
Choline, 39
Chromium, 22,31,49
Chymotrypsin,19
Cinnamon, 35
Cleansing Herbs, 63
Cleavers, 63
Coffee, 19,41,58
Complete Blood Count, (CBC), 59-63
Complete Protein, 10, 17, 23, 31, 37, 47, 58, 60
Complex Carbohydrates, 17
Copper, 27,33,35
Cranberry,12,13,25,27,42,56
Creatinine, serum, 46-47
Cucumber Juice, 39,51

Dandelion, 12, 13,14,19, 21, 22, 25, 26, 39,49,51, 56, 58, 60,62
Dairy,23
Detoxification, 58,61
Digestive Enzymes, 9,23

Echinacea, 62
Eggs, 12, 23
Elderberry, 45

Elecampane, 45
Electronic Stressors, 12, 58
Essential Fatty Acids, 10, 21, 41, 42
Evening Primrose Oil, 41,42
Exercise, 54
Fat Splitting Enzymes, 54
Fenugreek, 16, 21, 54
Fiber, 41, 58
Fish, 12
Flavonoid rich foods, 45
Flax Seeds, 21,41,42
Fluids, 17,18,41
Folic Acid, 12,18,27,31,35, 49

Garlic, 16, 21,27,35,54, 61,63
Ginger, 21,43,45
Ginkgo, 45,60
Ginseng, 12,16,17,22,23,25,29,43,54,56,58
Globulins, Total, 34-35
Glucose, 15-17
Glutamic Acid, 18
Glycine, 18
Gonads,16,22,33,46,47
Green Leafy Vegetables, 41,49
Green Tea, 21,31,35,58
Guggel, 58

Hair Mineral Analysis,19,35
Hawthorn Berry,31,33,45
Heart, 41,45,49
Heavy Metal Detoxification, 19
Homeopathy Revisited, 8
Horsetail, 29,58
Hydrochloric Acid, 12, 42,47, 62
Hypothalamus, 16, 17, 25, 29, 33, 36, 37, 41, 42, 43, 45,54,60,61

Inositol, 25,58
Intestinal Substances, 42
Iodine (kelp),29,36,39,58
Iron (Fe),48-49, 22, 26, 33, 35, 49, 56, 62
Iron rich foods, 49,60
Iron, salts, 49

Kava kava, 29,58
Kidney,12, 13, 27, 41, 51, 18, 39, 42,50,56,60

Lactate Dehydrogenase (LDH), 30-31

Laetrile,33
Lecithin, ,23,47,48,54
Left side nutrients, 48
Legumes, 23
Lemon Balm, 29, 36, 37, 43, 45, 54, 61
Lemon, in distilled or reverse osmosis water,33
Licorice, 9, 16, 19
Lipase, 10,17,48
Liquid Whey, 10,23,42,46
Lithium,29
Liver,14,16,18,21,25,29,48,49, 54, 56, 58, 61, 62, 63
Liver Detoxification, 21,54,62
Low Carbohydrate Diet, 16,21
Low Fat Diet, 16
Lungs, 45
Lysine, 12,13,45,58

Magnesium,9,13,17, 18, 23,25,35, 41, 45,
Major Organs and Glands, 6
Manganese,22,33,49
Meat, 12,23,60
Mental Stressors, 12,16
Methionine, 12,45,58
Milk Thistle, 19, 21, 26, 31, 33, 54, 56, 63
Mint Leaves, 41
Molasses, 49, 60
Molybdenum, 22,49
Mullein, 31
Multi-mineral complex, 50

Natrum Muriaticum, 43
Nettle, 9,10,18,39,50,56,58
Niacin (B3), 12,17, 21,27, 31, 35, 41, 43, 48, 54, 56
Nicotine, 58
Nucleoproteins, 19
Nuts, 12

Oat Straw, 9,18,35
Onions, raw, 21,54
Orotic Acid (B13),23,42,46
Orthophosphoric Acid, 12, 25
Ovaries,17,22,33,46,47

Pancreas, 13, 16, 17, 18, 29, 31,36,47,54,
Pancreatic Enzymes, 12,19
Pantothenic Acid, 41
Parasites, 62

Parathyroid,47
Parsley, 22,39,49,51,60
Passifloria,17
Pau D'Arco, 63
Peppermint,45
Phosphorus, 11-12,27,35,36
Pineal Gland, 27,41,47,54
Pituitary Gland, 13, 16, 21, 27, 47, 54, 56
Posterior Pituitary 17, 39, 41, 42, 50, 51
Potassium (K),40-41, 13, 14, 29, 39, 42
Potato Skins, 41
Poultry, 12
Primary Anti-Oxidants,63
Promethion, The, 27, 38
Protease, 10,17,23
Protein, Total 22-23
Proteolytic Enzymes, 51
Pulsatilla, 9

Raspberry, 50,56
Raw Bone Concentrates, 60
Red Clover, 9,17,39,50
Red Rice Yeast, 21
Rose, essential oil,17,33
Rose Hips,29
Rosemary,63
Rubidium,29

SAF Stress-120 Questionnaire, 12, 53, 58
Sage,27
Sarsaparilla, 43,63
Saunas, 17
Schisandra, 21,58
Seeds, 12
Selenium, 22, 63
Silica, 35, 43,63
Skullcap, 10,18,35
Sodium (Na), 38-39,29,39
Sodium Chloride, salt, 43
Spinach, 10
Spleen, 26, 27, 33, 35, 36,48,49,58, 60, 61, 62, 63
St. John's Wort, 23,29,39,58
Stomach,42
Stress, 54
Strontium, 17, 25
Strontium, salt, 18

Sunflower Seeds, 41
Super Oxide Dismutase, 35

Tea, 58
Testes, 17,22,33,46,47
Thalamus, 36,45
Thiamin (B1), 12
Threat of the Poison Reign, The, 27, 53
Thyme, 25,27,35,54, 62, 63
Thymus,13, 16, 17, 18, 25, 26, 27, 33, 35, 36, 48, 49, 58,61,63,62, 63
Thyroid, 13,21,35,36,45,58,60
Thyroxine (T4), 57-58
Triglycerides, serum, 52-54
Trypsin, 19
Tryptophan (5-HTP), 17

Uric Acid, serum, 18-19
Uva Ursi, 39

Valerian, 17, 54, 58
Vanadium, 22,49
Vegetables, 16,23
Vegetarian Diet, 18
Vitamin A, 14, 26, 35, 37,39,41,45,46, 58, 61, 62, 63
Vitamin B complex, 12, 16, 17, 26, 29, 31, 56, 58
Vitamin B1, 17,26,33,39,41
Vitamin B2,12,17,27,35,43
Vitamin B5,26,33,39
Vitamin B6, 13, 17, 26, 39, 41, 47, 48
Vitamin B12, 17,26,39,48,63
Vitamin B15,46
Vitamin B17,33
Vitamin C, 17, 29, 35, 41, 43, 54, 58, 61, 62, 63
Vitamin D, 10,37,39
Vitamin E, 14, 18, 26, 37,39,41,46,47, 56, 61, 62, 63
Vitamin K, 13,37

Water, Reverse Osmosis, (or distilled water) 13, 33, 39, 50, 61
Weight Loss, 12
Wheat Grass Juice,18,33
White Willow Bark,33
Whole grains, 12,16,39,41

Yarrow, 45
Yellow Dock,17,22,36,54,56
Ylang Ylang, 16,22,33

Zinc,12,27,31,41,61,62